Beyond Nurses Notes

A Journey to Choose Life

by
Mary M. Hale, RNC, MSN, SRN, SCM

CCB Publishing
British Columbia, Canada

Beyond Nurses Notes: A Journey to Choose Life

Copyright ©2008 by Mary M. Hale
ISBN-13 978-1-926585-12-3
First Edition

Library and Archives Canada Cataloguing in Publication

Hale, Mary M., 1940-
Beyond nurses notes: a journey to choose life /
written by Mary M. Hale – 1st ed.
Includes bibliographical references.
ISBN 978-1-926585-12-3
1. Hale, Mary M., 1940-. 2. Hale, Mary M., 1940- --Health.
3. Coronary artery bypass--Patients--United States--Biography.
4. Hysterectomy--Patients--United States--Biography.
5. Nurses--United States--Biography. I. Title.
RT37.H34A3 2008   610.73'092   C2008-907749-0

Cover design by Joto, age 5, one of the author's patients.

Extreme care has been taken to ensure that all information presented in this book is accurate and up to date at the time of publishing. Neither the author nor the publisher can be held responsible for any errors or omissions. Additionally, neither is any liability assumed for damages resulting from the use of the information contained herein.

All rights reserved. No part of this publication may be reproduced, stored in a retrieval system or transmitted in any form or by any means, electronic, mechanical, photocopying, recording or otherwise without the express written permission of the publisher. Printed in the United States of America and the United Kingdom.

Publisher: CCB Publishing
             British Columbia, Canada
             www.ccbpublishing.com

To my parents, Mary and Raymond Hale, who had me after trying for years "to just have one child who might make a difference." They gave me everything I needed, not everything I wanted, and prepared me for the sacrifices of life.

Acknowledgements

With all my gratitude to my physicians:

To Dr. Lynn Morris, M.D. and his team of cardiologists and surgeons at Albert Einstein Medical Center in Philadelphia, PA, who have heart. I asked for the very best and I received it.

It takes a village:

To my primary physician, Dr. Kenneth Hoellein, M.D., who insisted that I have a cardiac stress test pre-operatively, which I failed miserably and made me choose life.

To my surgeons, Dr. John Myers, D.O. and Dr. Justin Chura, M.D., who got rid of my cancer. And to Dr. Linda Bogar, M.D. who rebuilt my heart.

To Dr. Sumeet Mainigi, M.D., who paced me for life.

To Mary Beth Kingston, our Chief Nurse Executive in the Nursing Department at Albert Einstein Medical Center, who has been an example to us all, whether it be keeping vigil in the ICU with a family of a slain police officer or trying to get to the bottom of an altercation among patients and visitors. For her, caring is the cornerstone of her profession. As sure as the sun rises, her nurses are there to care for us.

To Colleen Connell, whose care and dedication in putting

together my first book "On Uganda's Terms," as well as this book about my returning back into the American profession of nursing, has been a joy to me as the author.

To June Lowe, RN, who hired me thirty years ago (while I was still in Uganda) at Albert Einstein Medical Center sight unseen, to work on her pediatric floor. She has served for me as a true example of what the spirit of nursing truly is and really should be. Her friendship has been invaluable to me over the last thirty years.

To my best friend, Dolores Connell, who has inspired me for 68 years, with her true concept of what it is to be a mother in every sense of the word. And to her husband, Tom, who is always there for all of us.

To my colleagues, Anita Bond, RN,C., Mary Kampf, RN,C., Ruth Noesner, RN,C., and Joanne Slutsky, RN,C., whose story contributions to this book make our teamwork a visible part of our nursing life.

To Bonnie Kaye, my friend and mentor for the last 25 years. She made me see the importance of choosing life and passing it on to others.

To Janet Mathis, my friend for 30 years, who used to warn me at night when trouble was coming to Pediatrics through the Emergency Room. For her sense of humor and instilling in me my positive attitude, I am truly grateful.

To the Nurses involved in the Visiting Nurses' Association, especially Bernice Green, who came twice a day to my home to care for me after my surgery. A big Thank You!

Last, and most important of all, to the Administration of Albert Einstein Medical Center for providing me the atmosphere to completely recover. I thank you and continue to spread the news that Einstein is a terrific hospital, with caregivers that provide us the atmosphere to choose life.

Contents

Preface 1
Introduction 3
Re-entry 4
Reciprocity Nursing 7
Tales from the Comfort Basket 9
  Why History – in Maternal Pain Management 11
  A Sign of the Times – Comfort Science 13
  Comfort for Whom by Joanne Slutsky, BA, RN,C 15
  Comfort by Anita Bond, RN,C 17
  Comfort from a Basket by Mary Kampf, RN,C 19
  Daddy Long Legs 21
  Fireworks Comfort by Ruth Noesner, RN,C 23
  The Godmother's Necklace 25
  First Toy 27
  The World of the Five Year Old 29
  John Henry by Joanne Slutsky, BA, RN,C 32
  Mr. Lemon 35
  Sad Pumpkins 38
  Short of Breath 40
  The Purple Dinosaur 42
  Conversation: Sir Sam Beagle Versus Bently Pitbull 43
  Warm Christmas Socks 45
  Love's Request 47
  Clifford Who? 49
  Nursing Exemplified by Bonnie Kaye, M.Ed. 50
Conceptual Model 53

Maternity Matters 55
Dedication 57
Happy Birthday! 58
Family Centered Maternity Model: AFRICAN STYLE .. 59
Ethical Options 61
Identity Dyad 63
Social Baby 64
A Picture is Worth a Thousand Words 66
Any Port in a Storm – The Blizzard of 2005 67
Breastfeeding: Successful or Unsuccessful 68
Close Call 70
Infection 24/7 71
Miracle Baby 73
Relaxation Breathing 74
Shaken Baby Syndrome 75
Social Service 77
Teamwork for Life 78
Twenty-four to Sixty-five 79
Relaxation Breathing for Two 80
Progress from Portugal 81
Length in Love 82
From Russia With Love 83
First Time Dad and Doctor 84
Boy or Girl 85
Remember Me 86
Rosary Beads 87
The Cord 88
Time Out 89
Do You Want the Book Back? 91

Brian's Song 92
The Saga of the Boarder Babies 94
This Time Is All You Have 95
Life Interrupted 96

References 99
Other Publications by this Author 100

Mary M. Hale

Preface

This book has been written twice – once to explain how my patients have made me the person that I am - and the second time, after I was a patient myself resulting in a quadruple cardiac bypass surgery with a pacemaker.

I have met all sorts of nurses and ancillary personnel during my six week hospitalization in Albert Einstein Medical Center, Philadelphia, PA. There are what I call "the hangers-on" who are only at a job for the money. Fortunately, these are few. Then I met the heroes, who do their daily duty in helping me to come back from a heart that would not start after a quadruple cardiac bypass.

My journey through this experience started with symptoms that necessitated me to go to the Emergency Room with CAT scans and various tests that showed that I was affected by a drug interaction. Then came a journey through a GYN visit, resulting in "abnormal cells" from a PAP smear and biopsy.

On the road to a hysterectomy, the abnormal PAP smear resulted in a failed cardiac stress test, as part of my pre-admission testing. One of the best days of my life resulted from a failed cardiac catheterization when my cardiologist stopped the procedure before causing any harm. What a blessing to meet people who know how to do their jobs well.

My primary physician would not compromise when I originally refused the cardiac stress test.

My GYN surgeon would not operate until I had my surgery to correct my damaged cardiac vessels.

My cardiac surgeon was a petite female who knew exactly what she was doing. I came through with flying colors.

Now for the "out of body experience" I had in the cardiac intensive care unit. From sleeping to periods of awareness, I found myself floating above my body and looking down to a scene of 5-10 doctors and nurses working over me. One was pulling off my soaked hospital gown, another nurse was starting a new IV site, another doctor shouted "Push D50 IV – her blood sugar is 41." A week later when I was stable, I asked my nurse to check my chart for a 41 blood glucose and she said it was there.

Part of my motivation for survival is that I had to finish the story that I began. I realized that choice is what makes us human and I chose life with a positive attitude. Nothing is black or white.

Mary M. Hale

Introduction

In my first book, "On Uganda's Terms," I described my life of ten years working in Uganda, East Africa – five years under President Milton Obote (1964-1969) and under the Ministry of Health when Idi Amin was dictator (1974-1979).

I wrote my first book thirty years after my employment with Uganda's Ministry of Health and fulfilled my promise not to write anything about Idi Amin until after he died (2003).

I retired from Albert Einstein Medical Center in Philadelphia, Pennsylvania, on June 3, 2006, after 27 years of service as a nurse in Pediatrics and Obstetrics. I can't help thinking about the demons that still haunt Africa – the recent violence in Kenya, one of the most stable nations in Africa, shows that poverty, corruption, and tribalism are far from cured (TIME Magazine).

After three decades beset by genocide, famine, AIDS, and wars, as obscure as they were endless, much of Africa is thriving. Often undercurrents of stunting growth and hurting its people continue. The outcome in Kenya, after the past election violence, may well determine whether Africa's renaissance sustains itself – or turns into another nightmare.

Re-Entry

After my escape from Uganda, East Africa in 1979, how was I going to re-enter into the American nursing profession after an absence of ten years?

I had experienced ten years of working for the Ministry of Health in Uganda during the most horrific of times, during the reign of dictator, Idi Amin thirty years ago. The spirit of nursing (caring) was always present among the Uganda Registered Nurses, even though supplies would come and go.

I can remember traveling sixty miles upcountry in a Land Rover with a patient in obstructed labor. We had no catgut suture for a cesarean section and had to travel to an upcountry hospital where they had the suture. We had to use dissolvable suture. If we placed metal clips, the patient would never come back for removal, so we used dissolvable catgut suture. Several of the women would come back annually with the metal clips embedded in their skin.

During Amin's regime, the Ugandan-Tanzanian War occurred, leaving most Ugandan hospitals without medication and supplies. We did the best that we could, often with nothing. With love and humor, we were industrious, creative, generous with our time, and honest. We begged for dried skim milk from the "Save the Children Fund" in London. We went from business to business in Jinja to try and get the linens and material to outfit the NICU in our hospital. We planted our own "Mwanamugimu" (you have fallen into good things) nutritional garden. We approached the Jinja Lions Club for money and materials to build our patient latrines to assist with our public health concerns.

Children who require hospitalization, no matter what the cause, present a unique set of challenges that require a special set of skills of those involved in their care. The ability to work connectively with families, collaborate with colleagues and specialists, ask the right questions, and recognize "danger signs" in a patient's changing condition is essential to insure optimal outcomes. Add to this the legal, ethical, and social aspects of care, and the need for a multidimensional approach to treatment becomes obvious.

After a ten year absence from American nursing, could I just step back into it effectively? I met a complex number of challenges addressing the science, technology, pharmacology, and the human factor that influence what I would be doing. Always to the forefront was my commitment to quality and continuing education.

Could I utilize my knowledge in a new practice setting, enhance the care I would provide, and best of all enjoy the satisfaction I experienced as I witnessed the difference it made?

I had to discuss current trends, research based practices, and any further possibilities in the care of hospitalized children. I had to return to the medical library at Albert Einstein Medical Center to restudy pharmacology. Medications were entirely different in England and Africa than in America. For example, Demerol was known as Pethidine. Often our medications in Uganda were from Russia and China as well as Great Britain. I studied for three months and then took a written and oral examination.

Adherence to standards of care and compliance with regulatory requirements all pointed me in the direction of prevention. The pitfalls that a nurse can face daily are relative to her involvement in litigation regarding medically related issues. Had I been reduced to a Nurse's Notes checklist?

The area in which I found myself was both sensitive and stressful. I thought of myself as a good nurse. Would I be able to defend the care? I gave good care. I was very conscientious and tried to keep up with the patient load assigned and often would go the extra mile. Our lives are very busy with new admissions, codes, and off the floor procedures.

I learned that the interpretation of the medical records is the key when the quality of care delivered comes under scrutiny. I found that nursing today in the United States is concerned with the legal and ethical implications, risk management, nursing charting systems, integrity, bioethical decisions, and malpractice.

One of the symptoms that is universal is pain. It means different things to different people. I had to return to history and my historical roots. I entered my study remembering that our assessment of pain is reflected in how much we can enter into the patient's world.

I felt the best way to communicate to the public what nurses actually are and what they actually do is by storytelling. The stories you are about to read are from my own personal experiences at Albert Einstein Medical Center. Several of my co-workers have generously shared some of their experiences as well.

Mary M. Hale

Reciprocity Nursing

Reciprocity nursing involves the patient and the nurse. The nurse gives treatment, medication, and supervision to the patient, but in return the patient gives the nurse an insight into their spiritual and physical well being or their distressed state. The nurse takes this information and makes it part of her and changes both the patient and herself by this exchange to choose life.

The stories that follow will show how I have been changed by each encounter. When the nurse opens up herself to the meeting of the minds, there are a lot of risks involved, which often result in counseling.

But the risks are well worth a better insight into the light and darkness of the patient's pain.

The names of these patients have been changed to protect the patient's confidentiality.

Sometimes the secrets that we hold within ourselves change us professionally and make our life magical.

Beyond Nurses Notes

Tales from the Comfort Basket

Beyond Nurses Notes

Mary M. Hale

Why History – in Maternal Pain Management?

History provides us with a natural opportunity to acknowledge milestones, celebrate achievements, remember turning points, and honor individuals of courage and vision who have made significant contributions. History gives us a chance to recognize enduring values and commitments and, by doing so, to rededicate ourselves to these principles.

At another level, history can be occasions for deeper reflection. Even those most optimistic and upbeat would acknowledge that the progress of pain management has not always been smooth and that its forward direction has sometimes been difficult to discern. Historical inquiry may be helpful in discovering positive trends amid the confusions of the present. A broad historical perspective with scientific input can help us shrink specific disappointments to size and show them in context as only temporary setbacks. Historical case stories may be helpful to teach us useful lessons about successful strategies used in pain management in the past. They may assist us in identifying patterns and deeper continuities beneath the surface shifts of maternal pain management.

At yet another level, history may provide new insights into the difficulties of change, whether of social realities, attitudes, or behaviors. It allows us to perceive deep structural impediments, identify blind spots, and analyze social forces and cultural trends over which we have little control. At the same time, historical study shows us that despite the difficulties, change is possible, given dedication, organization, and persistence in caring for mothers and infants.

Mary M. Hale

A Sign of the Times – Comfort Science

For the past two years in maternity, we have been identifying comforting strategies and processes of comforting in conjunction with our pain management skills. But, comfort is a very elusive state.

It is no longer acceptable to us for the mother to "bear the pain" of a hospital experience. Comforting is provided in response to patient cues; it is patient-led. The mother presents us with an evident patient need. Responding to the need of the mother in pain is nurse-controlled.

Pain is what the mother says it is; it is the signs of distress on the face of the patient as observed by the caregiver and her verbalization.

A conceptual model evolved as we worked together in attempting to reduce and eliminate pain. We concluded that pain reduction came about by caring, comfort, medication, and diversion.

By writing stories, the caregivers on Maternity hope to reach the following objectives:

1. To understand more about pain and the comfort measures that we can take to eliminate pain, along with pain medications.
2. To understand more about the interaction between developmental level stimuli and distraction.
3. To tailor our assessment strategies to the mother's developmental level, personality style and to the situation.
4. To have an on-going historical record of pain management techniques written by maternal care-

givers, not only for our own review; but, as an orientation tool for our new caregivers.

We have found that comforting strategies are particular to special behavioral states. Ongoing nursing research has resulted in "The Theory of Comfort," which may be outlined as follows:

"Comforting is embedded in nurses' work and occurs as a normal and integral part of nursing care. The nurse assesses the patient and, in response to the patient's cues, to situational clues, or to an expressed need, identifies an appropriate comforting strategy.......Thus the role of the nurse is to assist the patient to maintain endurance and support the individual until the suffering is resolved."

"The Science of Comforting"
by Janice M. Morse, RN, PhD.
Reflections, 1996.

Mary M. Hale

Comfort for Whom
by Joanne Slutsky, BA, RN,C.

Not too long ago, a new patient care program was introduced on the Pediatric floor. It was not invasive, it did not measure anything; it did not analyze or deliver anything and yet it benefited both the patient and the staff. It is the Pediatric "Comfort Basket." The next question is "Comfort for Whom?"

Why do we say this? Because since its arrival, there has been some ambiguity about who derives greater benefit from it.

Part of Pediatric nursing involves many unpleasant procedures. Along with the joy of seeing most of our patients recover, we also have to deal with the many invasive and often unpleasant procedures to advance them to the recovery stage. One of the worst of these is lead chelation.

Lead chelation, besides involving the daily venipunctures for lead levels, requires frequent I.M. injections. The medication cannot be given intravenously due to potential problems with cardiac arrhythmias. Intellectually, all the nurses caring for the child are aware of this. What it does emotionally to both of us is another story. Of course, we carry out the necessary injections as professionally as we can manage, frequently hugging and reassuring the child afterwards about what a good boy or girl they were and that they were not being punished for anything.

The "Comfort Basket" enables us to give something besides emotional care, something that is much more tangible for children – "goodies!"

We all remember a little three-year-old boy who had to endure the painful BAL and CaEDTA injections. Another nurse and I would carry the basket in with us when it was time for his injections. He would get so enthralled in choosing his next little present, that it momentarily distracted him from what was about to happen. Of course, it is not to say that he anticipated his injections with great joy; but, maybe it was able to diminish their importance.

Both the other nurse and I were thrilled to be able to have a "Comfort Basket" to offer him. This leads us back to the initial question – "Who is comforted by it?" Is it the nurses who offer it or the patients who receive the little gifts?

The question still needs to be decided, but, I secretly think that the answer may be both.

Comfort
by Anita Bond, RN,C.

Comfort according to Webster means "to allay grief or trouble; to console, cheer, gladden. To ease a body or mind, or to provide solace or consolation."

Some time ago, a co-worker of mine, Mary Hale, introduced the idea of a "Comfort Basket" to the Pediatric Department. When she provided the concept of the "Comfort Basket," my mind flashed back to a very personal incident that occurred when I was seventeen years old.

Due to a congenital deformity of my spine, I was forced to spend some time in a hospital. Having just undergone a spinal fusion, life was anything but comfortable. Fortunately, there was one nurse that I will never forget. She surely fit the stereotypical "Angel of Mercy." This was before the time of Emla Cream and PCA pumps. My nurse understood one very important thing--something few people understand. She understood the importance of diverting physical and emotional pain through gentle "hands on" care, and "something to do."

I was the typical teenager. All of my friends were having fun. I was having none. This nurse spent time with me each day, listening to my problems, and there were many. She provided support when I was discouraged. She offered things to take my mind away from the pain and frustration of not being like everyone else. She gave me books, crossword puzzles, and a very funny pair of prism glasses.

I finally left the hospital over one month after I was

admitted. Imagine that today. I finally could resume the "normal" life of a teenager spending time with my friends.

I will always remember that devastating time of my life. Though I never saw her again, I will always remember and love Miss Dunkle.

The items found in the "Comfort Basket" provide diversion from one's pain, either physical or emotional. I have long known that pain medication was not necessarily the only remedy for pain. Offering an item from the "Comfort Basket" diverts the discomfort our small patients are going through to something more pleasant.

A recent incident on the floor proved to show just how important the "Comfort Basket" can be.

Two small children were admitted to the Pediatric Department after ingesting an undisclosed amount of a medication belonging to a relative. It became necessary to do hourly blood work on these two little people.

Every hour the blood stick brought weeping and wailing, and flailing hands and feet. No amount of explanation, or attempting to prepare them, helped them to understand why they had to be stuck so often.

By late afternoon the lab work revealed that the problem was resolved.

After the last specimen was drawn, they are each presented with a "Barney" party hat and a lollipop. Their smiles literally lit up the room. I knew, once again, the importance of the use of a "Comfort" item from the "Comfort Basket." I knew they had been comforted in their pain, and I finally made two new friends.

Thank you, Mary, for the comfort of having a "Comfort Basket" in the Pediatric Department.

Mary M. Hale

Comfort from a Basket
by Mary Kampf, RN,C.

I vividly recall the psychological agony of my childhood trips to the dentist. My mother would attempt to calm my anxiety before each visit by discussing what to expect, then she would remind me of the ring I would receive for being "a good patient." I remember the thought of the gift ring as reassuring. It also strengthened my resolve. Even as a child, I remember trying to live up to my perceived part of the bargain. I wanted to earn that ring. These rings were shown to peers in the school yard, and they were respected as a badge of courage. They were worn until they fell apart, long after our finger had turned green.

Now, as an adult, my dentist invites his patients to take a flower from the vase at the end of each visit. I look forward to this modern day acknowledgment that I did what I needed to do and was being recognized.

Being acknowledged or recognized for a difficult task is what these gifts are all about. If someone modifies their behavior to be an easier patient during treatment because of the acknowledgment they have learned they will receive in the end, then all the better.

This is an elegantly simple idea that, over the course of time, I had forgotten.

So many times we go to outside conferences and are reminded of these good ideas but fail to act on them. The Pediatric Department of Albert Einstein Medical Center can thank one of our staff nurses for bringing home to our unit an idea she heard at a conference. That is the idea of "The Comfort Basket."

After a treatment or procedure is performed on one of our patients, they are invited to choose a gift from our "Comfort Basket." After a long stay, some of our children have quite a pile of these little gifts. These gifts are even more important because many of our families struggle to get bus fare to visit their children, much less have money for the luxury of a gift for that child.

These little gifts are our way of acknowledging what our patients are going through. They also help to divert attention from all of the negative things associated with being in a hospital. I have also observed some of our older children being very brave during a procedure as they try to "earn their badge of courage," even though a gift promised is never withheld because of behavior during a procedure.

After I've offered the verbal sympathy or hugs that follow a painful or difficult procedure, I must confess that it helps me as much as it helps my patients to be able to give them a tangible thing to recognize their struggle. As I analyze the situation, it even helps give closure to these painful situations because of the rhythm that develops with use of "The Comfort Basket." If the child is able to walk to where we keep the basket, we use this time to further allow the child to calm before picking their gift. If they are bed-bound, they often calm down while I go to "The Comfort Basket."

Either way I have found this basket to be a useful tool and all-around great idea that has worked its magic on our young patients.

Mary M. Hale

Daddy Long Legs

Evan, age five years, was hit by a car while rollerblading. The car, literally, had to be lifted off of his left leg. The result was a fractured left femur with multiple abrasions to his right ear, face and right shoulder.

Evan was his parents' "precious one"; he was their only son. Early in infancy he had to have a diaphragmatic hernia repair, as well as repair surgically for malrotation of his large intestines. During his first few months of life, he had been in and out of hospitals; now here he was back again at five years of age.

Evan was with us in Pediatrics from August 13th to his discharge on September 7th. His first and foremost problem was the pain – skeletal traction, portable x-rays, pin care, neuro-vascular checks. All were new and scary to Evan.

What could we give Evan from our "Comfort Basket" that would accompany his pain medications and be a diversion for him? Evan would not drink and we gave him a drinking cup shaped like a yellow Crayola crayon. He would not touch it at first; then he began to weaken. He enjoyed a simple game involving his Crayola crayon drinking cup and did eventually begin to drink.

His skeletal traction suspended him in space; he tended to shift his alignment and he had to be repositioned. During the night, he began to have nightmares. One member of his family was always present at his bedside and we would work with the family member and Evan to ease his fears.

He began to be more and more dependent on his family member and our staff. Self-help development was on hold. One staff nurse brought in "Daddy Long-Legs" to hang from his traction. It was a cardboard "Scarecrow" with two foot long tubular legs filled with bubble gum, ending with cardboard sneakers.

Evan let the "Scarecrow" hang on his traction for a few days without comment. Then his play skills took over – he felt the toy and even tried to open the legs to get at the bubble gum. You could see him thinking when he was finally able to chew small amounts of the balls of bubble gum. He asked his mother and one of the caregivers – "Can I use bubble gum to paste my leg back together?"

"Not yet, Evan. Maybe by the time you grow up and become a bone doctor that will be the treatment of choice." Evan went home to a loving family; but, is not back to rollerblading yet.

Mary M. Hale

Fireworks Comfort
by Ruth Noesner, RN,C.

Whenever we worked July 4th weekend, there were always a few fireworks accidents. I received an admission on Saturday night. He was thirteen years old and he had found a firecracker in the backyard and it exploded right in his hand. He lost part of his thumb, all of his index finger and a part of his second finger. There was also a deep wound in his palm, which had been repaired.

Hand surgeries are painful and he was on a Patient Controlled Analgesia Pump. He was on I.V. fluids and his injured hand was in a vertical sling, elevated on a pole. To understand him a little better you have to know part of his medical history. He has ADHD (Attention Deficit Hyperactivity Disorder). We have found that the worst thing you can do to these children is to require them to be still and alone.

No one came to the floor with him when he was admitted. His family left the hospital while he was in the recovery room. We placed him in a semi-private room, but he had no roommate. When he fully recovered from anesthesia in the middle of the night, the scenario would be his injured arm is in the vertical sling on the one side and the other arm is connected to two different pumps, which both alarm when he bends his elbow.

My challenge for the rest of the night was to hope that morning arrives without the disconnection of the I.V. lines and further injury to his postoperative wounds.

I spent most of the night from 2 a.m. to 7 a.m. in that room with him. We checked out the "Comfort Basket" for something that would be age-appropriate and diversional for him. He chose a Beeper Bubble Gum Pack and playing cards. He was delighted with his prizes, but especially that they were his to keep. He did offer to share with the nursing staff.

We played cards off and on for the rest of the night. I would tell him what I had to do and he would be calling out frantically in less than two minutes – very pleasantly and politely, but still just as demanding.

We played cards, thanks to the "Comfort Basket," but most of all, we reduced his pain, as well as all the stressors of hospitalization.

Mary M. Hale

The Godmother's Necklace

Janet had been a patient on Pediatrics since she was three years old; now she was sixteen. I happened to meet her in the hallway where she had just visited her three-week old godchild. Imagine, our Janet, a Godmother.

She had originally come to us thirteen years ago via Fire Rescue after a house fire. She was covered with soot and blisters. In the years that followed she had multiple admissions for asthma. Our goal with Janet, as well as all our other children, was to reduce the incidence and severity of children's acute pain, whether it be postoperative, medical procedures or as a result of trauma.

Throughout her hospitalizations, we could see her altered development related to the stressors of hospitalization. Adolescent stressors are a loss of independence, separation from her peer group, altered body image, as well as the various procedures.

During her last hospitalization, we assisted her in maintaining her independence by participating in and cooperating with her care. Her contact with peer groups was facilitated; sometimes we thought the phone was permanently attached to her ear!

Near the end other hospitalization for asthma, she really began to demonstrate a positive body image through positive statements and behaviors. What could we give Janet from our "Comfort Basket" that would foster her new positive adolescent behavior and act as a diversion during some of her procedures? We brought the "Comfort Basket" into Janet's room and let her choose what she wanted from the basket.

She chose a gold colored necklace and as I sat down to help her put it on she spoke about all the diversions available to her age group: arts, crafts, hobbies, board and card games, video games, T.V. movies and reading. But the most important thing of all was to allow time for her to discuss concerns, fears and ask questions.......to listen. Her life as a teenager in the hospital had embodied choices, privacy, and comfort.

There, in the hallway, when Janet was visiting her godchild, I told her how great she looked standing up and dressed in the latest fashion. Usually on the night shift, she was in bed and wore the "universal" fashion of the hospital gown.

She held onto my arm and pulled on the gold colored necklace around her neck and said, "I still have the necklace from the "Comfort Basket."

Mary M. Hale

First Toy

Joseph, age eight months, was admitted to the Pediatric unit for the second time in his short life for eczema, which covered his body from head to toe. Upon his admission, nobody accompanied him, nor did he have any toys with him.

We had been discussing altered development related to the stresses of being hospitalized. For an infant it would be very stressful to be separated from his parents. We placed him in an isolation room with a bubble top crib for safety. Being in such a room gave Joseph little environmental stimuli which he desperately needed.

What would be done to make Joseph's stay with us a more pleasant and comfortable one? Our "Comfort Basket" had a large plastic bubble push toy; the bubble was filled with small colorful balls which jumped around when pushed. Besides giving him his pain medication, nurses are aware of the importance of diversion. When the toy was put into the crib with Joseph, the response was amazing.

One of the first comfort measures for Joseph after his pain medication was a bath. He was gently dried; a lot of dried flaky skin came off his body onto the towel. His skin was flaky from head to toe. The eczema on his head was so severe that much of his hair had fallen out. After his bath, he was dressed and wrapped in a crib blanket and put to bed with some soft radio music.

As you left Joseph's room, the sound of the rolling ball could still be heard. His response to the toy was so dramatic you could not help but wonder if this was his first toy. A short time later the noise subsided and

Beyond Nurses Notes

Joseph slept peacefully into the next day with his new toy at his side, waiting for him to start a new day.

Mary M. Hale

The World of the Five Year Old

What is "The Comfort Basket" and what is it doing in Pediatrics? 'The Comfort Basket" is a collection of diversional toys, books, puzzles, etc appropriate for pain management for children of all ages. These diversional items are used with pain reduction medications to bring comfort to each child or adolescent. "The Comfort Basket" is kept in the medication room to remind each nurse of its value, along with the pain medications.

Deeshawn was a normal five year old - full of vigor, sure of self and had attained personal mastery in a number of observable ways. Five-year-olds will let you know that they are competent young people, able to attend to many of their physical needs, verbalize their thoughts and feelings, and socialize with other children and adults. Five-year-olds acquire the knowledge and skills to function with considerable independence in a familiar environment--but a hospital environment--that's another story. A diagnosis of asthma and pneumonia with chest tightness and pain left Deeshawn not so sure of himself.

Even though the basic personality pattern of the five-year-old is established, a child will continue to develop and mature in whatever environment presents itself. The child's personality continues to make itself visible. Deeshawn's talents, temperament, and ways of handling the demands of everyday life were evident, and it was possible for people who know the child to get a glimpse of the emerging little man.

Physically, five-year-olds are more in control of movement and enjoy active and energetic play.

Deeshawn's physical stamina and growth were increasingly evident, and so was the child's intellectual growth. During the disease process, we have to guide five-year-olds by providing stimulating materials and new experiences. Along with our observations of the physical process, we observe the child's work, which is play. Five-year-olds are expert observers and like to describe objects. The child begins to move from understanding me now, and here to you there and then. There is increased understanding of the meaning of time. Humor emerges in the form of telling jokes and planning unexpected surprises for the nurse and family. In asking Deeshawn the question, "Where do dreams come from?" responses included: "They're little pictures," or "The moon sends them." The child of five is still egocentric and everything that is perceived or felt seems to be common to his whole world. Everything is external and real. Emotions are strong at his age. Fears and anxieties are usually temporary and concrete and are manifested in thunder, sirens, darkness, solitude, nightmares, and the very strong fear that mother will leave and not return. Children should be comforted and assured that they are safe.

Play is important in the world of the five-year-old. According to some theorists, play is early life-hood education at its best Play is, among other things, an act of discovery. As children play with the blocks from "The Comfort Basket," they learn about number concepts, relationships, and the properties of our physical world. Some children like to see their words in print. They may tell a story, describe an experience, or draw their own pictures. If play reveals the nature of a child, so does the creative expression that emerges from the use of paints, crayons, markers, water-colors and other materials.

Deeshawn was asked what he was drawing so diligently He said that he was drawing a picture of God. The nurse told him that no one really knows what God looks like and he stated "When I am done, they'll know what He looks like!" Children of this age are likely to believe that inanimate objects are alive in the same way that humans are alive. The sun and flowers may have faces and animals may wear clothes.

Just because they are hospitalized does not mean that children do not need the time and opportunity to explore the possibilities that exist within their developing minds and bodies. Sensitivity to the needs of children allows us to share on the work and world of the five-year-old.

Hospitalized five-year-olds are allowed to choose what they want from "The Comfort Basket," along with their pain medication. They want to be open and honest with the adults in their lives about their pain. They want to share, because they want feedback and enlargement on their own experiences. Five-year-olds are beginning to understand the excitement of intellectual discovery and are beginning to see adults as resources for expanding their mental world. The world, seen through their eyes, is an infinitely exciting, mysterious, and challenging place to discover and enjoy - pain free.

Truly, the pediatric nurses can give and give to these children remembering the old proverb, "It is hard for an empty sack to stand upright." Deeshawn cried when he said good-bye to the nurses on Pediatrics. He held tight to his grandfather's hand, as he disappeared around the corner to the elevator.

John Henry
by Joanne Slutsky, BA, RN,C.

"John Henry was a steel-driving man." Those were the words that went through my mind when I first met John and Henry. But in my case, John Henry turned out to be steel driven boys. Let me explain.

In May, 1996, we were informed that the pediatric floor would be receiving two motor vehicle accident victims. One, Henry, was a nine-year-old, and the other, John, was a sixteen- year-old. The boys had been riding on a motor bike when it was struck by a car careening around a corner. Both boys suffered right femur fractures; one fractured midshaft and distally and the other fracture was proximal. Both boys were in the operating room for approximately two to four hours and both boys would be wearing external fixator devices for quite some time. This required dressing changes twice a day; six pin sites for Henry and eight pin sites for John.

The two young men were well medicated prior to the pin cleaning While that may have lessened their actual pain, it did not alleviate the emotional discomfort of seeing steel rods going in one side of their leg and coming out the other. The surgeons, well aware of the initial psychological impact such a sight would have, sent both boys back from the operating room with the devices well wrapped in kling bandages.

When we first removed the bandages from John's leg, Henry, in the next bed, was able to see how the "Erector set" was built around his friend's leg. Henry's reaction was immediate and unstoppable - he leaned over his bed rails and vomited. John, the older boy, did not go as far as Henry, but he was extremely apprehensive and vocal about his dislike of having any part of his leg or the device touched.

John and Henry's fears and apprehensions were understandable and appropriate. But, except for medicating them, which was done, and reassuring them that we would be as gentle as possible, which we were, there was not much else we could do. I spent a great deal of time with both young men and their parents, explaining the procedures and attempting to lessen their fears. Then I remembered our "Comfort Basket."

What could that "Basket" hold for a pre-teen and a teenager? It had coloring books, crayons, bubbles and slinkies, rattles and baby toys. Then I saw them, a collection of rubber-jelly finger puppets! John and Henry had to have their pin sites cleaned twice a day. They were promised a finger puppet for each cleaning. By the end of five days, they would have enough for all ten fingers. I guaranteed them that by the time they had a full puppet hand, the pin care would be much less onerous. Instead of scoffing at the idea, both boys enthusiastically agreed.

Those finger puppets did the trick! Yes, they continued to be medicated and yes, they continued to voice their concerns, but that now was somewhat mitigated by the anticipation of receiving additional little puppets for their collection.

By the third day, both John and Henry were assisting with the pin cleaning. By the fifth day, Henry said, "Remember when you told us that it was going to get better? Well, you were right and when I'm home, I'll be able to do my own pin cleaning."

The boys were very possessive of their finger

puppets. Once somebody had come into their room while they were down at Physical Therapy and had "thoughtfully" cleared the bedside table of extraneous materials. Upon their return to their room, there ensued quite a vocal discussion of "who had taken their puppets." Luckily they were found in the bedside drawers.

John and Henry, our steel driven boys, took those finger puppets home with them. Both the external fixator and those silly, little rubber toys became symbols of their triumph.

Mary M. Hale

Mr. Lemon

The "Comfort Basket" is a diversional method of reducing pain in pediatric patients. It is used as adjunct therapy, along with the administration of pain medications. Toys/diversions are administered by the nurse and/or caregiver in a timely manner.

Bobby, age 11, was admitted to Pediatrics post-operatively after a tonsillectomy and adenoidectomy. He had the "dreaded" I.V. and was not drinking. Bobby was receiving I.V. medications for his pain but was very anxious. He was physically tall and lanky for his age, and never far from his Mother. Bobby's Mom was post-op one week from a hysterectomy and was spending the night with Bobby in the hope of his discharge the next afternoon.

Bobby had great difficulty in getting to sleep in a strange bed. We had recommended to the family to bring in familiar objects to remind the patient of home and family. We discussed with the Mother several appropriate interventions and involved his parents in his care. Nothing seemed to work. It was then the "Comfort Basket" went to work. We had one plush toy-- a "Mr. Lemon" pillow with a smiley face.

Our experience tells us that appropriate activities for a child of Bobby's age would be arts/crafts, hobby activities, board and card games, videos, TV and movies, as well as reading.

We are well aware of the Goals of Pain Management in children:

- reduce the incidence and severity of children's acute pain (post-op, medical procedure and trauma).
- educate children and their families to communicate about pain.
- enhance the child's comfort and increase the child's and the family's satisfaction with pain management.
- reduce post-operative complications and reduce the length of hospital stay.

We had to combine pharmacologic and non-pharmacologic options when appropriate. "Comfort" has been defined in Webster's College Dictionary (1991) as,

"To soothe, console or reassure; bring solace of cheer, to comfort someone after a loss. To make physically comfortable; relief in affliction; consolation or relief. A state of ease and satisfaction of bodily wants, with freedom from pain and anxiety."

Our problems with Bobby also involved his altered development related to the stressors of hospitalization. School age children's stressors are: separation from family, separation from peer group, decreased opportunity to achieve mastery, boredom and parental knowledge deficit.

Working with Bobby's Mother, we both understood the importance of diversion. Bobby bonded immediately with "Mister Lemon". This was a round plush pillow colored and shaped like a lemon with a big smile. Mom stated that she thought it was the toy's smile. For myself, I'm not

Mary M. Hale

so sure; it could have been Bobby's love for lemonade. Early in the morning he started to drink - Lemonade, of Course!

Sad Pumpkins

Sam was four years of age and had never been hospitalized before with asthma. His parents smoked at home, "always in the basement; sometimes outside the house." The smoking was thought to be the trigger for Sam's hospitalization.

At first Sam was so sick, requiring two I.V. Pumps, fluids, medications and bed rest. His games were on hold for awhile. Then he was able to walk and move to the playroom. His favorite word during the first few days of hospitalization was "owie." No matter who asked Sam where his "owie" was, he would simply point to his heart. It was passed on the next shift during report about the "owie," so that we could get to the bottom of this.

Everything was examined, prodded, listened to, and talked about. The little boy took on a sad face and no amount of diversional activity could take away his sadness. Until one day a resourceful nurse told Sam that he would be home in time to pick out his Halloween costume and go out with his friends and parents "Trick or Treating" in his neighborhood. This was all that Sam needed to hear - he would be home in time for Halloween.

For the next few days, while he was getting better, Sam would make his daily trip to the playroom full of fun, games, puzzles, etc., and always drawing and coloring a pumpkin.

Then Sam heard he was going home. It was early evening before his parents came to pick him up from the Pediatric floor.

One of the nurses gave him a pair of Pumpkin

Mary M. Hale

glasses - two pumpkins with the eyes cut out so that Sam could see where he was going. The glasses were a little big for Sam, but so was his smile. He was heard saying, as he went down the hall with his parents, "I think I'll just wear these "Pumpkin" glasses for Halloween!"

Short of Breath

Nijay was eighteen months of age and had a past medical history of asthma. He was admitted to Pediatrics this time with a cough, increasing temperature, otitus media, plus rhinnorhea for two days at home. His shortness of breath worsened overnight, requiring oxygen therapy. His parents had left him alone for the night.

His birth history had been a three week stay in our NICU with increasing respiratory difficulty at 37 weeks of gestation. His permanent residence was with his great-grandmother and father, where he stays with his mother. His Dad is involved in his support and care.

This time in Pediatrics, physicians had diagnosed Group "A" Hemolytic Strep. His physical environment included a bubble top crib, side rails, and isolation. As we all know, familiar sights and sounds have a comforting effect on toddlers. He certainly knew how to wave "bye-bye" and shook his head "no." He had been busy learning new things at home before his hospitalization. His attention span was short with a preference for his own toys, which his parents had forgotten in their rush to provide medical care for their son.

Besides the physiological stress of his multiple problems, he also had the separation from his parents, as well as the inappropriate stimuli of the various tests during his admission. He was refusing everything as far as fluids. Then we had an idea about the possibility of utilizing something from 'The Comfort Basket."

Should we choose a toy or perhaps something to persuade him to drink? We had small water canteens shaped like houses, airplanes and stars. Using the distraction technique we put apple juice in the airplane water canteen, played with the airplane and the child for awhile and left the canteen in the crib. He still continued to cry as we closed the isolation door. I stood outside the door and watched. The TV was on with its diversional music. He explored the objects in his bed by banging, throwing and dropping, and then he tasted them. When he came to the airplane, he looked at it and drank from the plastic straw attached to the canteen.

All this activity took time, and by the time 2 a.m. came, the security officer had called that his parents were in the lobby and wanted to come and visit him. Since he had been asleep when they left at 9 p.m., they were surprised by all the activity that had gone on since they left. They had returned with his favorite teddy bear and found him holding his "dee" drink. He certainly had developed a sound that had meaning. Toddlers do not misbehave on purpose; they understand "no" but will still need us to direct their attention to another more appropriate activity.

The successful recovery of Nijay can be directly attributed to his oxygen therapy, antibiotic and pain medications, diversional activity, along with a caring, loving family and nursing staff who utilized a firm, direct approach with Nijay.

When we said "bye-bye" to Nijay he held as tightly to us as he did to his parents and cheered us all by saying "dee-dee." We all miss him.

The Purple Dinosaur

Brittany is an adorable girl with dark, curly hair and brown eyes. I remember the first time she saw me and how fearful she was. She was alone in the hospital, away from home and familiar surroundings.

I went into Brittany's room and placed her in a stroller for transport. During the trip downstairs, she was very quiet and still. Before she went into the room for her procedure, she looked at me and appeared to have a sad expression. I gave her a reassuring smile.

Brittany was very cooperative during the entire procedure. The technician awarded her with a plastic watch with beads inside that moved around and a sticker that read "You're a SuperStar." The child's smile was like a beam of sunshine.

During the entire trip upstairs, Brittany was more interactive with others and made sounds that seemed like pleasurable noises. Upon our arrival upstairs, I took Brittany to her room. I then went to our Pediatric Unit's "Comfort Basket" and selected a purple dinosaur drinking canteen. When I gave Brittany the canteen, she grinned from ear to ear. Never again that night did she appear quiet or withdrawn.

As busy as any shift in the hospital can get, it is essential to give our young patients "comfort" items to alleviate, if only temporarily, their anxiety and fear associated with a hospital stay.

Mary M. Hale

Conversation:
Sir Sam Beagle Versus Bently Pitbull

Christopher was a lively ten-year-old that had been stopped in his tracks by a bout of acute pharyngitis. He was admitted to Pediatrics early one morning around 1 a.m. His official diagnosis was left peri-tonsillar abcess and he was not happy. He also had a very high fever and was very irritable.

Both Mom and Dad had accompanied him to the floor and all were oriented to the patient room facilities and the pediatric protocol. Still, Christopher was not talking. His throat pain was an obvious problem. We gave him his pain medication and waited.

Christopher also had a history of asthma, but his lungs were clear at this time. Mom and Dad both answered "no" to the questions about "Any Pets at Home?" I also asked them at this time if Christopher would like a roommate if we did admit a boy around his age. Christopher finally opened up and said "Yes - when?" We explained to the family that as soon as there was an appropriate boy admitted, Christopher would have a roommate. He seemed pleased. Then Mom and Dad left for the night. I made frequent visits to Christopher that night - "Please leave the light on." "Roommate yet?" All his questions told of his loneliness. It was his first time away from his family and home.

Then I thought some diversional conversation would help with his light sleeping. I asked him if he would like some company with storytelling. I could see by this time the pain medications were working and he was more verbal and grateful for company. I told him I had a dog by the name of "Sir" Sam Beagle. Story after story of Sam's antics poured out - interrupted by many questions from Christopher. Then with his parents' answer to the "pet" question in mind, I asked Christopher if he had a dog. And the answer was very surprising. "Yes, Bentley Pit Bull." An hour went by while Christopher told me the stories about his dog and the joy he brought into his life. Then Christopher began to nod and I knew that sleep would not be far behind. Our friendship has been cemented by our love of animals. Now, when I asked him on a Scale of 0 to 5 what his pain was – he said zero.

I told him in the morning before breakfast that the lady-nurse coming on to take my place had a farm with sheep and that he could ask her all about sheep. They would have a good day.

The next night when I came on for the night shift, I found out that Christopher had been discharged that afternoon to go home. It seems that he had talked to his day nurse about her sheep and had forgotten his pain.

His antibiotic therapy and pain medications around the clock had done the job – plus the diversional conversation!

Mary M. Hale

Warm Christmas Socks

Christmas is a warm season with cold feet for little infants. Jonathan was here for Christmas and New Year's Night. This was the day of his circumcision and he was a little irritable.

Jonathan had been transferred from the Neonatal Intensive Care Unit to Pediatrics to complete his fourteen-days of antibiotic therapy for meningitis. When I took care of Jonathan he was twelve-days-old.

Keep the infant free from pain and keep him warm-we learn-but sometimes we forget the infant's feet. My mother used to teach me when I was a child that if your feet are warm, your whole body is warm.

Pain medications were given prior to the circumcision - so very important to relieve the coming discomfort. Bright colored soft toys were placed close to him, as loving thoughts from his family.

We know that pain is whatever the child says it is or in the case of an infant - whatever the nurse observes - especially the quiet facial expression of physical distress. The facial expression was the most consistent behavioral indicator of pain in infants.

The "dollar" store is a favorite place for some of the anonymous donors and nurses to search for additions to our "Comfort Basket" for our pediatric patients. Warm Christmas socks are often found in great supply around the holidays. Infant sizes are no problem; some of the very tiny infants have warm socks that go all the way up to meet their "onesies." One common denominator among all the infants - from the preemies on up - is the sigh of contentment - after their warm Christmas socks are on and their pain medication is given.

Mary M. Hale

Love's Request

Natasha Love was admitted to Pediatrics with a diagnosis of intussusception. She was only three years of age and very outgoing and verbal. Her orders read that she was only to have I.V. fluids and nothing by mouth for a while.

Her diagnosis of intussusception is a prolapse of a segment of the intestinal tract (the intussusceptum) and subsequent telescoping of that segment distally. Her history of vomiting and intermittent colicky abdominal pain had taken its toll on Natasha and her mother. Now in the hospital, confirmation and management took time- plain films and barium enemas- which were looked at as the gold standard for diagnosing and treating intussusception. Her mother remained with her throughout the whole hospitalization. Managing Natasha's pain and diversional activity were another problem.

Our "Comfort Basket" on Pediatrics has a number of "good things" for three-year-olds. Her first day was spent with hair care on an Afro-American teenage doll. The weekend was filled with coloring and paint with water-type books and stories.

But, the most important thing to us now was dealing with her hunger, since she had progressed to clear liquids only. She would run to the nurses and search our pockets, asking if we had "Doritos." At night she could be heard calling out to her mother for a cookie. Three year old explanations of why you cannot eat do not go very far, but the diversional activities did help somewhat.

Finally, after the third barium enema to resolve the intussusception, a colonoscopy was done to remove a polyp and after a 24 hour period of observation, Natasha was discharged.

She was seen going down the hallway to the elevator holding on tightly to her mother's hand and waving a bag of Doritos.

Mary M. Hale

Clifford Who?

Clifford had been on Pediatrics for four days prior to my being assigned to his care. He was a sixteen-year-old adolescent on Pediatrics with a diagnosis of deep vein thrombosis, secondary to Salmonella infection from his pet iguana.

Day after day his Heparin I.V. treatment and bed rest continued. Clifford has a loving family that brought him many diversional activities. The "Comfort Basket" provided a "Seek and Find" word game for his age.

Now a little about Clifford's history. "Clifford, Who?" I asked and when I was given his last name. I said, "I know him." Sixteen years ago I had taken care of Clifford in the NICU (a thirty-one weeker) with Beth Cephus as my preceptor. How do I remember him so well? We had a great deal of difficulty keeping his colostomy bag on under the warmer bed. He had his colostomy anastomosed at three months of age, according to his mother.

When Clifford was born, his mom was fifteen years of age and now she looks like his sister - and that's alright with Clifford and his mother.

Nursing Exemplified*
by Bonnie Kaye, M.Ed.

There are the some people who have the misfortune of spending much too much time in a hospital due to chronic illnesses that require repeated and/or long term hospitalizations. To us, an outstanding nurse is not just a friendly greeter, but rather a lifeline to sanity and good health.

My son, Jason, was born in 1982. From the time he was three weeks old, he was ill. He was presenting gastro types of illnesses like chronic diarrhea and vomiting, but after months of testing by his GI specialist, no verdict had come forth. He was stumped. Jason continued going to the hospital for abscesses that appeared on different parts of his body until he was diagnosed by an infectious disease specialist with a disease called Chronic Granulomatous Disease, a very rare immune deficiency in the white cells. There were only 500 people in the county that had this x-linked disorder which was handed to mostly sons by their unsuspecting mothers—like me.

As a child, Jason had three different liver abscesses within a two year period which resulted in long-term hospitalizations as we—patient and doctor—learned that long-term antibiotics were NOT the way to resolve the problem—only surgery would take care of it. Those hospitalizations when Jason was 6 and 7 lasted up to five months. I would move into the hospital and be at the mercy of flea-biting mattresses provided for the mothers on a fold-out chair.

The pressure and the anguish of living through those

Mary M. Hale

days were horrific at best. Exhaustion became my middle name, and my own health certainly suffered while caring for my son. There was one nurse who stood out above all others—Mary Hale. I had the luck of meeting Mary during Jason's toddler stage when he was admitted to the hospital on a number of occasions. Mary exemplified nursing because she looked at each situation holistically. She knew that if I was there taking care of my son, I would need nourishment to keep up my strength. She cooked for me on a number of occasions knowing that by midnight, I'd be hungry after a long day. She saw the mental stress that I went through, and this was part of her concern as well as Jason's health.

While other nurses would put on the full lights to get Jason's temperature in the middle of the night waking both of us up from desperately needed rest, Mary would always come in the room with a flashlight, allowing both of us to sleep and get the rest. We were always so relieved when she was on duty.

Mary was never a sitter—she was a doer. She would roam the floors checking in on all of the patients, especially the crying children in pediatrics. It was rare for a parent to stay overnight, so when the lights were out, the children were crying for their mothers. Mary always would go in and comfort the child, and those kind words went a long way. She even would come to the hospital dressed as a clown on her day off to entertain the children, always bringing a comfort basket filled with toys and goodies.

My son remained a patient on that pediatric floor until he became an adult. His last hospitalization on the pediatric wing took place when he was nearly 17. That's when he insisted that I leave the hospital and not stay with him. He wasn't a baby anymore! The only way I would leave and have peace of mind was to know that Mary was there checking in on him. At that age, he wasn't too thrilled about the flashlight, but he sure loved Mary as if she were his family. He also had a sense of comfort knowing she was there.

I tragically lost my beloved son, Jason, in November 2005 at the age of 23. He was on his way to becoming a teacher when he died from pneumonia which had been incorrectly treated medically. My life will never be the same because there is a part of me that is still in such unbelievable pain. It is very hard to look back over his life to this day without feeling my greatest sense of loss and sorrow. But if I have to look for the one good thing that came out of his tragedy, it is Mary Hale. This woman exemplifies what nursing should be—kindness, compasssion, caring, and dedication. Never was heard a discouraging or disheartening word. Follow-up was the order of the night with Mary. You didn't have to ask her to do something—she knew automatically what to do. Mary Hale is nursing at its best. I felt very excited that I was able to nominate her for a prominent nursing award a number of years ago from the Pennsylvania Association of Nurses. It was my honor to be there when she picked it up after they honored her. Thank you, Mary, for being a role model for those in your profession.

* This story was added by the editor.

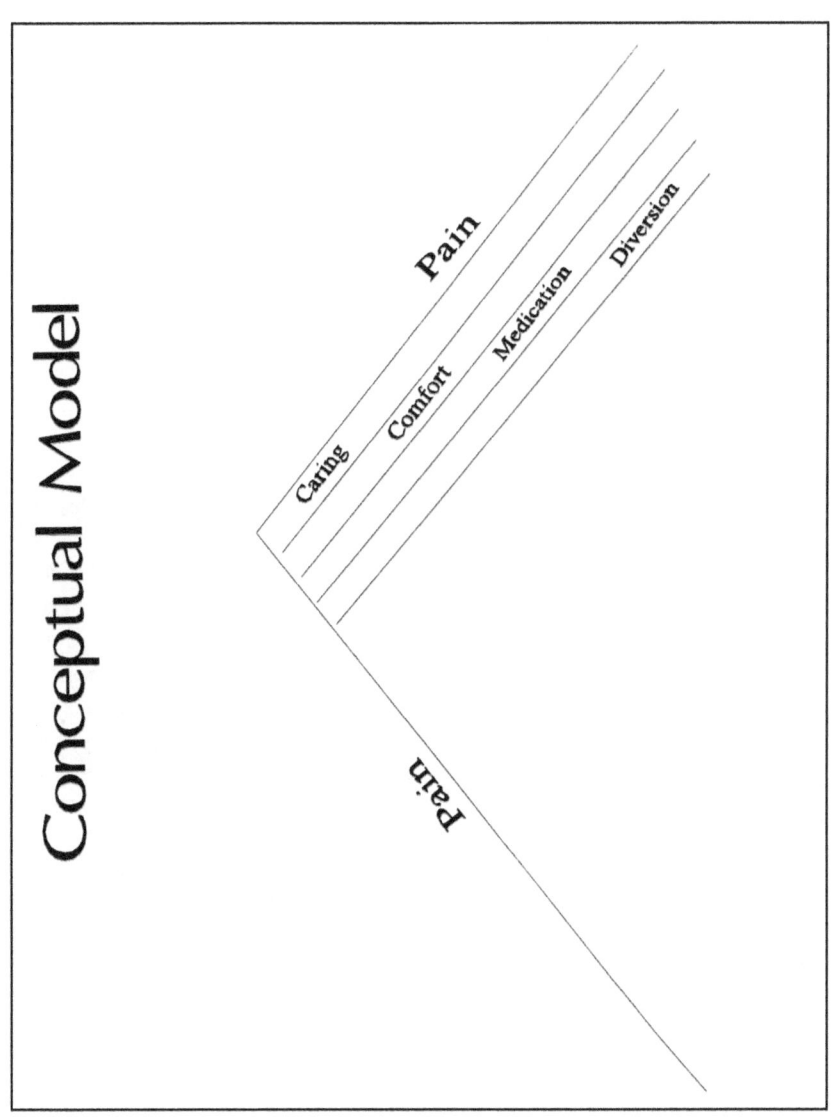

The Conceptual Model
As pain increases; pain will decrease with these four options.

Beyond Nurses Notes

Maternity Matters

Beyond Nurses Notes

Mary M. Hale

Dedication

To All Maternity Nurses

Everywhere, Who Realize

That Their Profession Is

REALITY With The

Sound Turned Up!

Happy Birthday!

Dear Newborn,

This is an open letter to you newly born little one. You have come through a lot in just being born. Now you have your whole life ahead of you.

You will now enter into a partnership with your parents. You will begin to understand the lessons from the past, the realities of the present and the likely consequences of a decision for the future.

You will be filled with good intentions. You will find yourself to be a disturber and an awakener at the same time. You will have the ability to "dream great dreams". You will brighten our lives, as we go through all of our life's circumstances.

You will find your entire life revolves around two emotions or whatever you call them....**LOVE** and **FEAR**. We live our whole lives trying to figure out how to embrace them or run from them.

It's up to you to find out what works for you to be happy.

And, by the way, Happy Birthday!

Mary M. Hale

Family-Centered Maternity Model: AFRICAN STYLE

When I first went to Uganda in East Africa thirty years ago, Maternity care not only included the physical, but social, spiritual, psychological, and economic dimensions as well (Phillips, 1997). One could never separate the family from the newborn.

Nursing the Mother and baby as an interdependent pair-dyad or couplet is ideal for family-centered maternity care. What is best for the Mother and her baby is our first concern.

Scenarios such as continuity of care, ongoing teaching, and Mother-infant bonding are all contributing factors in the parents becoming more confident with their parenting abilities (AWHONN practice monograph, Mother and Baby Nursing). The Mother-Baby Dyad promotes an active environment for the transition to the home environment.

In East Africa, there is no compartmentalization of families. The welfare of the Clan is uppermost in their minds. The midwife shares the teaching with each relative beginning with the Mother and the Father of the infant.

Each person in this world has the right to help in healthcare, which promotes wholeness in the body, mind and spirit. We, as healthcare professionals, must continue to learn and think in different ways to improve healthcare. A healthy culture begins with each person and is enhanced through self-worth, partnerships, and systems support.

The cost of delivering quality care in Maternity lies in our willingness to create a safe place to learn collectively and seek diversity. To acknowledge mystery, to share thinking, and listen to the thinking of others, to be surprised and to honor the presence of each person's humanness, no matter what culture, that is body/mind/spirit in transition, never static.

Mary M. Hale

Ethical Options

Patty had been our Pediatric patient since she was 2-1/2 years old with Sickle Cell Disease. Now she was 24 years old and having her first baby, but only 4-5 weeks gestation. Her admitting diagnosis on our Maternal/Infant Unit was her sickle cell pain.

She called me on the Pediatric floor to come and visit with her. I came to visit her and discovered her ulterior motive. She stated that she suffered very much in her life and wondered if she had her baby if he or she would also inherit the sickle cell pain. "Should I have an abortion?" she asked me. What should she do?

I told her she should meet with her parents and sister to discuss her options. I also told her that I could present her choices, but she was the ultimate decision maker. She understood.

During the next several months, I heard by way of the grapevine that she had been admitted again and again for her pain management. Then, all of the sudden, her delivery date was here. Jonathan came into this world in the cold of winter. I went to see him in the Nursery and couldn't believe what I was seeing. There asleep in the nursery crib was the most perfect little body I had ever seen. Since Dad had sickle cell trait and Patty was sickle cell positive, what were the chances that young Jonathan would also test positive?

She told me his blood work had to be sent out of state and she was awaiting the results. I wondered what my choice would have been if I were in her position. Would I take the chance? Would my faith be strong enough?

Later during another admission, I saw her in the

hospital lounge awaiting the delivery of her pizza. I asked her about Jonathan, and she said his test came back negative and that she was enjoying him so much.

A year later I heard from her relative that she had died in bed with Jonathan at age 26.

Mary M. Hale

Identity Dyad

A seventeen-year-old teenager was admitted to our Maternity Unit of Postpartum mothers. She delivered a small baby girl and the Labor and Delivery Unit identified the baby with two bracelets. With the various activities and procedures that we have to do with the baby, the ID bracelets are checked numerous times daily.

While checking the baby during the evening care, the bracelet was discovered missing. The nurse questioned the mother, examined the bassinet, baby and mother's room. The mother was notified of the importance of finding the missing bracelet. The staff discussed the options among themselves. Perhaps she kept it for her "baby book." Another possibility was that she had given it to the father of the baby or as she stated, she just "threw it away."

The staff nurses in Maternity give care to mothers and infants in dyads. We nurse both Mom and baby together as a unit. Often, we are in the Mother's room demonstrating feeding to a new Mother. It is at this time the identity of Mom and infant are checked. The staff stressed the importance of the missing I.D. bracelet responsibly during the various shifts. Consistency was our theme.

The teenager finally admitted that she gave the baby's bracelet to her new boyfriend. Need I say more?

Social Baby

When it's feeding time in the Nursery, some newborns eagerly await their first feedings while others sleep. There are multiple variables that determine how well each infant will take their formula.

In a study of observation concerning the readiness of the infant to feed, we found that if the nurses talk to the baby and each other, they feed even so much better.

Tanya had a reversal of a tubal ligation last year and now she had a Down's Syndrome female infant. In helping Tanya to bond with her infant after the shock at her birth, we had a lot of ethical dilemmas. Tanya felt she let her second husband down with his first baby - a Down's Syndrome baby. We worked with Tanya from the moment she spoke with her obstetrician announcing that she had delivered "a very sick baby." I was with her, and we discussed her options. I demonstrated a feeding technique that works almost all of the time, namely, talking with the Mother as I feed her infant. We discussed her daily schedule.

Daily bits of information regarding her care and the care of her infant were taught, encouraged and laughed at with good humor. As we discuss what will go on at home during feeding time, she could see how well her infant took the formula, burped and then took more formula.

It was during our talks that I discovered that Tanya was a corrections officer with shift work. She stated how she needed to find a job with nights and weekends off, so that she could be with her baby. Unfortunately, she did not have any family members that she could trust with the baby.

I knew of a job opening with the city in the Air and Noise Pollution Department that provided the kind of schedule that Tanya needed and I referred Tanya to them.

We, as Maternity nurses, respond with care, compassion, integrity and respect – old ideas that work!

A Picture is Worth a Thousand Words

The Staff Nurses in the Maternity floor admit Mothers whose infants have to be admitted to our Neonatal Intensive Care Unit.

Dawn had a cesarean delivery of a tiny baby boy, who had grunting respirations at birth. Dawn had an opportunity to look at him for a few minutes, and then she transferred to our Maternity floor.

She was very drowsy from her morphine infusion. We checked her frequently and each time she asked for her infant.

As we turned and repositioned her and taught her relaxation breathing, she asked what happened to the picture of her infant. I called the NICU and spoke to the infant's nurse, Lisa. Lisa said that she had spoken to the Mother before her transfer to our floor.

Earlier, six nice photos of Dermot had been taken with the digital camera in the NICU. The mother was beginning to get restless and stated that the morphine drip was not working anymore. She asked again for the infant's photos.

Later that night, Lisa came up from the NICU with the photos and the Mother was just delighted.

Her pain decreased and she went to sleep with her infant's photos in her hands.

Mary M. Hale

Any Port in a Storm – The Blizzard of 2005

The snow just kept coming. Every time I looked out the window during the day, I kept thinking about how I was going to get to work for the night shift (11pm to 7am). I prepared for the worst – getting to work on our Maternity Unit.

I went back to bed for my nap before I started shoveling. Suddenly, there was a fever of knocks on my front door. Six children, ages 6 to 13 years old, were standing there with shovels and brooms ready for action. "Can we dig you out?" they asked. Was I ever glad to see them!

I called the Maternity Unit and informed them that I was on my way. I packed my things into the car and the engine started right up. I warmed up the car and the kids began pushing me out of the parking space. They cheered and clapped as I turned the car around and headed to the hospital.

I stopped the car and opened the driver's door and shouted out to them in my best Elvis impersonation, "Thank you. Thank you very much!"

The nurses who had worked the previous twelve-hour shift were glad when I arrived, so they could finally sleep within the hospital for another eight-hour shift in the morning.

"Any port in the storm," shouted one of the patients holding her newborn infant, "Thank God it's ours!"

Breastfeeding: Successful or Unsuccessful

What is the determining factor in the success of breastfeeding? There are many variables that we are taught over the years.

Both quality and quantity figure into the equation for successful breastfeeding. The quantity of time that the infant is with the mother is of the utmost importance with regards to bonding and breastfeeding. Trish was fourteen years of age and intent on breastfeeding. She also wanted to be "on the go" doing what fourteen-year-olds do.

The night shift is sometimes ideal for testing both the quality and quantity of breastfeeding. The quiet undisturbed time of mother and infant together can never be recaptured early in the infant's life. But, on the day shift, our lactation consultant is our guiding light regarding helpful hints that have proven useful throughout the years. Ellen Prince, our lactation consultant, provides the quality part of the breastfeeding equation.

For example, Trish was a Temple football fan. When we demonstrated the breast-feeding infant "football hold," she really started to catch on. She really never thought of holding her infant in that position. We reviewed the safety factors with her and looked at her "latch score." Use of the individual categories, such as breaking the latch, giving bottles, pacifiers, etc. help to remind us of what is to be taught as we are supervising the mother and infant.

When the staff nurses are orienting to our postpartum maternity, we all have the great privilege of orienting with

Ellen, our expert in lactation. Things do change over the years and Ellen is educated on all the new ideas and techniques. We are grateful to her for sharing them with us. Trish, our fourteen year old, is very, very grateful as she says "Way to go, Ellen. Thank you."

Close Call

It is always interesting when we have a physician as a patient on our Maternity floor. Twenty-eight year old Paula was from Colombia and had given birth to a baby girl. This was her first child. Mother was breastfeeding with formula supplementation after the breastfeeding.

Paula was a very good first time breast feeder. She would feed for thirty-five minutes. Later she told me (just one time) that she had placed the infant in the bassinette and slipped into the bathroom for a moment. She heard the infant start to choke and went quickly to the infant's side. She discovered the infant dusky in color and not breathing. At this time, she grabbed the infant and ran down the hall, holding the baby over her head and shouting "My baby's not breathing!"

We calmly took the infant from the mother and went to the nursery to suction the infant and administer oxygen as needed. Paula accompanied us to the nursery and was reassured by the pediatricians and nurses. The infant "pinked up" nicely and settled in the nursery for close observation and monitoring.

It was at this time that I really became familiar with Doctor Paula and her history. She had a history of sudden infant death syndrome in her Colombian family. Two of her sisters, we found out later, had close calls with their infant and toddlers. This mother confided in us that even with all of her medical training, when it came to her own infant's safety, she couldn't remember a thing except to get HELP for the close call.

Mary M. Hale

Infection 24/7

It seems that infection in Obstetrics is on the rise. More and more pregnant women are coming to us with sexually transmitted diseases.

Ursula was one of these women, whom we will always remember. Prenatally she had a diagnosis of syphilis, with a very high titer. She was very compliant with her treatment. At the time of delivery, she had reduced her titer four-fold.

When Ursula came to us postpartum, she had a fever reaching 104 degrees. She was started on one IV antibiotic and gradually increased to triple IV antibiotic therapy. When I entered her room during the night shift, a pair of sad eyes looked at me from under the covers. I introduced myself to Ursula and proceeded to sit down with her and inform her of the night shift routine.

Ursula's assessment came first, then the transfer of the baby to the nursery for the routine assessment and bath.

Now it was her time alone once the baby had been taken to the nursery. My questions came out of concern. What did she have for dinner? Was it hot? Her assessment came, along with conversation about her beautiful baby and, of course, congratulations for all of her hard work during her delivery.

Then it was her turn, and the questions just flowed about the CAT scan of her pelvis due in the morning. Did she have to fast after midnight? What was this "contrast thing" she had to drink before the scan? She would not consent to another IV site and this "control" issue had been going on for the last 24 hours.

I explained to her the seriousness of the CAT scan to arrive at a definitive diagnosis. Then I approached the reasoning behind the IV access for her safety. She then consented to the IV insertion.

In the early morning, she had her breakfast and fed her baby. She said she was feeling much better. As we saw the escort take her to the CAT scan, I couldn't help but think of all of the infections that have not yet been detected and the sorrow they will cause in countless lives. But, on the other side, there is hope with IV antibiotic therapy and caring conversation.

Mary M. Hale

Miracle Baby

Glenda was a 40-year-old second time Mom. Her other child was 21 years of age and quite a young man in college. Glenda had a history of tubal ligation five years ago.

The report of her medical history was quite extensive. It included obesity, congestive heart failure, osteoarthritis, gastro esophageal reflux, chronic hypertension, knee surgery, and a tonsillectomy.

Her daughter, Grace, weighed in at seven pounds and fourteen ounces. She was quite a surprise after the tubal ligation five years ago. Glenda, her mother, could not have been happier. In addition to having a beautiful daughter to raise, Glenda also realized that she had a caregiver for her later years.

Mother and baby are in the process of bonding together. The infant is feeding well and gaining weight every day.

Babysitters will not be a problem.

Relaxation Breathing

Many times we have patients in Postpartum who are on narcotics for their pain management. Kyen was a twenty-five year old first time Mom, who had a Cesarean Section operation for failure to progress in her labor.

When she first came to the floor, she was managed on a regulated Morphine Pump, which she regulated herself. After a day or two, she progressed to oral medications. This patient had convinced herself that the oral medications would not work. She demonstrated this behavior by numerous calls to the nurses' station for help and a "need for more medication."

After collaborating with the physicians, the Staff Nurse decided she was a good candidate for our "Relaxation Breathing" exercises. A nurse sat by her side and demonstrated the various relaxation techniques; i.e. relaxation of the upper and lower extremities, visualization of the ocean waves going in and out, listening to the sound of the waves with the help of a compact disc with sounds of the ocean waves, heavy rain, a summer's night and a running brook.

With the introduction of the compact disc, the relaxation breathing exercises became more real. Based on our experiences, we found that the pain medications worked quicker and Kyen concurred.

Mary M. Hale

Shaken Baby Syndrome

Every month or so, the newspapers shout out a headline about a recent "Shaken Baby Syndrome" case. So when we speak to our new mothers about the continuance of care, we ask if they have enough help at home to care for the baby/babies.

Short tempers are part and parcel with the "feeding, crying, and wetting cycle."

Jackie does all of our Hearing Screening Tests prior to discharge. As she goes around to all of our Mothers, she carries a small plastic case with a rubber brain floating inside. When she shakes the case, it causes the brain to snap back and forth. This simulation shows the new mother how shaking a baby can lead to serious and often permanent brain damage.

Jackie taught Bria, a new mother, to be patient in trying to figure out what her baby needs. She encouraged her to stay calm in assessing the baby's needs. First, see if the baby is too hot or too cold. She could then check the baby's diaper and/or feed the baby. After burping the baby, she could offer a pacifier or toy.

Jackie stresses environmental factors such as taking the baby to a quiet room and holding the baby against the chest and walking or rocking the baby gently. When Bria gets home from the hospital, she could also take the baby for a ride in a car or stroller. Bria suggests that sometimes an infant swing can help to soothe the baby to sleep.

For the Mother, if the baby's crying really becomes bothersome, we suggest a short break, so she can practice some slow and deep relaxation breathing. We

also recommend a bit of exercise, listening to music, or reading to help the new mother to relax.
But most important of all, Bria knows to ask for help!

Social Service

Some of the gifts that have shaped my personal and professional growth are: appreciation, humor, challenge, intellectual growth, flexibility, and privilege.

All of these gifts have bound nursing together with our Social Service Department in the person of Gwen Tate. Our days are full of listening, empathy, healing, awareness and persuasion. Some patients tug at our heartstrings more than others.

Partnerships are essential to plan, coordinate, integrate and deliver healthcare across various cultures in our hospital.

I remember one particular patient, who had just delivered a female child. The husband was observed striking the Mother. We intervened and advised the Social Service Department. Later, we observed the Mother hitting the bed and telling the infant to be quiet. We also learned that both parents had wanted a boy. We discussed this situation with Social Services and the physicians.

The collaboration of the physicians, nurses, and the Social Services Department allows us to continue to learn and think in different ways to improve the delivery of healthcare.

Each person involved is accountable to communicate and integrate his/her contribution to healthcare in our community comprised of all nationalities.

Quality exists where shared purpose, vision, values and partnerships are lived on a daily basis.

Beyond Nurses Notes

Teamwork for Life

In was early in the morning when Tiffany was admitted to our floor after a spontaneous vaginal delivery of a baby boy. Debbie was her admitting nurse. After assessing the patient, Debbie got her a cup of tea. When she returned to the room, she found the patient restless. She examined her and found that the patient was bleeding and had expelled a large clot.

The nurse called for help. We called the physicians and gave the sedation. A new I.V. site had to be started, since the patient had pulled it out in the elevator. We gave the I.V. fluid, along with medications to contract the uterus, after the physicians had examined the patient.

Vital signs and blood work followed but, most important of all, safety issues and comfort for the patient were of highest priority.

The patient slept for a good four hours, and we checked her frequently. Later that morning, when the Nursery Nurse brought the infant to the Mother, she awakened to his cry. The look of love on her face cannot be described, as she took him into her arms and said "God bless us, everyone!"

Mary M. Hale

Twenty-Four to Sixty-Five

Our staff ranges in age from 24 to 65 years. We have found that successful approaches to leadership are rapidly shifting towards a better way of working. Our work is based on teamwork and community that seeks to involve others in the decision-making. It is strongly based on ethical and caring behavior that attempts to enhance the personal growth of staff while improving the care and quality of our working environment.

We seek a delicate balance between conceptual thinking and a day-to-day focused approach. We are filled with good intentions. In striving to understand others, we learn to empathize with them. In our society today, we understand that self-awareness strengthens us. Awareness also aids one in understanding issues involving stress and values. It lends itself to viewing most situations from a more integrated holistic position.

In an effort to convince others, rather than coerce compliance, I was sitting in a Mother's room after demonstrating how to feed her infant. The door was open just enough to hear the call bell.

One of the newly admitted patients walked down the hallway and peeked into the room. She then asked the nurse sitting at the Nurse's Station if I was the infant's Grandmother. The nurse asked Who-What-Where and then laughed and said it was the patient's nurse. I told my patient what the woman had said and she laughed and said, "I guess the old-fashioned way might be misinterpreted."

Beyond Nurses Notes

Relaxation Breathing for Two

Rolanda was a 21 year old and delivered her first infant, a girl (8 lb. 4 oz.). She was extremely anxious when she got to her room on our Post-Partum floor. Her husband accompanied her with all of her belongings.

He looked worse for the wear. He had been up for 48 hours awaiting the delivery. When I gave his wife her pain medication, I taught her relaxation breathing to help her sleep.

I noticed him as I taught her the breathing and visualization. He was very attentive as he breathed in and out in time with his wife. He had sat in the chair next to her bed and as he focused on letting the tension go from his arms and legs, and I knew I was going to be in big trouble. He seemed to be settling in for the night, making himself more and more comfortable.

Finally, I had to remind him that he had to leave for the night and come back at 10 a.m. for visiting all day.

As he reluctantly left, he muttered something under his breath. When I asked what he had said, he simply stated, "I'll have to do that relaxation breathing again when I get off driving my SEPTA bus!"

Mary M. Hale

Progress from Portugal

Olga, 20 years of age, was a first time Mother who had just emigrated from Portugal. Milo came into this world at 7 pounds, 6 ounces and very hungry.

He had been conceived in Portugal and was just an American for two weeks before birth. Mom had carried him in Philadelphia when the temperature was in the high 90's this summer. Their little apartment had no air conditioning and no fans.

Her pregnancy had been complicated by a choroid plexus cyst, noted at 19 weeks by ultrasound, and resolved at 23 weeks of gestation. Otherwise, her recovery was uncomplicated except for the heat.

She came from a community in Northeast Philadelphia that banded together to help Olga and her family.

They went to the community center and arranged for fans to be delivered, compliments of the community center. The room air conditioner was paid for in part by the father of the baby and his friends.

Both parents are now enrolled in English language classes, taught by nuns at a local high school. Her husband has a possibility of a job.

While in the hospital, care was entwined between Nursing, Social Services and Interpretive Services.

Mom had told us prior to discharge through the interpreter that she was glad Milo would grow up speaking English with "No trouble," she said.

Length in Love

Most of our Mothers of our newborns always ask for the weight and length of their infant right after birth.

The weight of the infant is taken at the time of birth, but the length is done later on admission to the Nursery. It is placed on the identification card on the bassinette, where it becomes the topic of conversation during visiting hours.

Tanya just delivered her first girl, after four boys. She thought the girl was shorter than her boys, but the baby's length was not filled in yet on the bassinette card.

While doing my rounds at night, I asked her the usual questions. She answered, but I felt there was something wrong. I asked how her care was and then she let me have it. She stated that she was a college graduate and had much experience with breastfeeding her four boys. Now a girl came into their lives and she thought she was short. In the morning when I went around to see how the breastfeeding went, I brought the tape measure. She didn't say a word. She just watched what I did. After I measured her child, all 18 ½ inches of her, I wrote the inches on her identification card and told her what her length was.

Now she said she could rest well. She knew her infant was shorter than all of her boys at 21 inches. But something she said to me will always stay with me. "It's the small things in life that matter." Just the fact that someone remembered to tell her the length of her baby girl meant so much to her.

Mary M. Hale

From Russia With Love

Maria was 27-years-old and just had her first live baby. She had a Cesarean Section because the baby's cord prolapsed and she was on medication for high blood pressure.

I did not know what to expect when I went into her room to introduce myself. I had heard that she was in America for the past three years and knew very little English. A Russian interpreter was expected the next day to help with teaching and discharge planning. Social Service had to be involved. The infant's father had died of a heart attack several months before the baby's birth and Maria had no family members here in America.

Little Ludmilla was the best baby in the Nursery. She rarely cried except when she was wet or hungry. I had to remind her mother to breastfeed her every 2 to 3 hours to help decrease her jaundice.

As I got to know Maria, I found her shy about her knowledge of English. Through testing her with various questions that she would have to answer numbers, time, etc., I found her more and more anxious to speak slowly in English.

She relaxed more when she heard that the translator coming tomorrow would help her fill out the birth certificate information.

When the night was over and the sun came up, I told her how well she did with speaking and getting her ideas across to the various staff members.

I told her that I didn't think we would have done as well if we were patients in Russia.

First Time Dad and Doctor

Bob is a second year resident in obstetrics. He and his wife are from Poland and they immigrated here to America a few years ago. Now they were waiting their first child. The baby is a girl according to the ultrasound scan and her name is Julia. All await her arrival: physicians, staff, relatives, and especially her parents.

On April 25, 2005, Julia arrived at approximately 3 p.m.; a normal delivery without any complications. Julia weighed in at almost eight pounds. During the couple of days that they were in the hospital, Bob stayed in a private room with his wife and newborn baby girl. All the nurses were giving Bob hints on the various short cuts to a full night's sleep. One of the nurses stated that he really should know about babies, since he delivers them as an obstetrician.

He stated that he just delivers them and then hands them to another professional with that specific expertise. We all laughed and proceeded to show him how to swaddle Julia. Most infants, we have found, settled much better when wrapped tightly. It probably reminds them of when they were comfortable in their mother's womb.

Bob practiced and practiced, so he would impress his wife. After demonstrating to her, she said, laughing, "I'm not impressed. I know you too well!"

Mary M. Hale

Boy or Girl

Some parents yearn for a boy after four girls. Who knows what was said to Maria after her ultrasound. She heard what she wanted to hear – a boy!

The purchases and showers all favored the birth of a boy. All her girls awaited his arrival and they all had jobs lined up for him to do when he got older. And so the lists began. The first list was for his name. That was on hold until they all saw him and decided if he looked like a Matthew, Mark, Luke, or John. He would be named after one of the authors of the New Testament.

Maria's labor started early and she came into our Labor and Delivery room. A couple of hours and a few pushes later the baby arrived. What a surprise for everyone – a girl arrived without any complications. She was perfect in every way.

The next request (in the middle of the night) was for the name book. Mom searched until she found what she was looking for – her name was Mary Magdalen.

Maria's tubal ligation was on hold until next year, when she would try again for the boy.

Remember Me

Every so often we have an ante-natal patient on our Post Natal floor. Renee' had a three year old at home and was here with us on bed rest due to her infant's 33-weeks gestation and premature labor contractions.

The contractions had gone off for now but on the Evening Shift she felt sick after eating what her relative had sent in for her on this very hot, summer day.

After I checked her at midnight she finally fell asleep. We did all of our assessments, vital signs, fetal heart rate, etc. all at one time. I then had time to talk with her about her upset stomach pain.

She had said she was ready to try some tea and toast, which finally felt good. As we talked, I assessed her chest and breath sounds, since she had a history of asthma. Her lungs were clear and then I began to think that she looked familiar.

In our conversations, I learned that she had been my patient ten years ago in Pediatrics with her history of asthma. By morning, she was ready for a jelly donut!

Mary M. Hale

Rosary Beads

Penny was a first time Cesarean Section delivery who had been raised in Haiti. She arrived in this country two years ago and now had Henre', her newborn son.

I had taken care of Penny on her first night post-operatively. She was on a morphine drip with I. V. fluid. Penny slept most of the night. She held onto her rosary beads during the first night. In the morning we brought her newborn son to begin breastfeeding.

The second night she was taking narcotic pain medication pills. That night was uneventful and the breastfeeding went well. She was given her pain medication routinely with great relief.

On her third and last night, she rang the call bell and was found wandering the hallways. She stated there was a "heavy energy" in her private room. She felt a presence of a young woman, who came near and touched her clothes. She could not sleep. Two obstetricians came to see her and prescribed non-narcotic pain medication. They then wrote for a psychiatry consult for the morning.

In the meantime, we changed her into another private room near the Nurse's Station. I sat with her teaching relaxation breathing so she could finally go to sleep. She confided in me during the breathing exercises that her rosary beads had broken and when she repaired them the "Our Father" bead was missing.

She commented further that she had to have a relative bring in her new rosary beads so she could have her "blessing" again and peace of mind. I just listened.

The Cord

Clanna was 27-years-old and had 5 pregnancies, but only this infant survived. She had a baby girl, 7 pounds and healthy.

I worked with her all night teaching about feeding her infant and taking care of herself. Early in the morning she called and I went into her room.

She asked me what that wet thing was coming out of the baby's stomach. I explained that was the baby's cord and that was responsible for the baby's nourishment while inside the womb. She stated that it was wet and purple. I explained that the cord would dry up and fall off in couple of days.

She looked at me and simply said, "I don't believe you."

If you know another explanation, I'd like to hear from you!

Mary M. Hale

Time Out

Nicole was a 36-year-old registered nurse, who worked in our Medical Intensive Care Unit. She had a repeat Cesarean Section and had developed an amniotic emboli. She went from the Operating Room to the Medical Intensive Care Unit as a patient.

Three days later she was transferred to our Mother and Infant Unit. I had the opportunity to talk with her the first night she was with us. While we were evaluating her pain level, I asked her what it was like being a patient on the floor that she worked. She thought for a few minutes and then said her first concern was for her privacy, but she said she soon got over that. She stated that she hardly had any time to herself. Her numerous blood specimens, Doppler tests for decreasing circulation, and vital signs left her little time for resting.

For several nights her baby was cared for in the Nursery. We scheduled her care so that her various procedures were combined to allow her time to sleep. We scheduled her pain medication so that her pain level was decreased substantially during the night.

We explained the importance of keeping the Sequential Compression Devices on both her legs to promote circulation. Her subcutaneous Heparin injection was scheduled every eight hours, also for prevention.

She stated that after a few days she could relax and not look at the level of her I.V. fluids.

Today she is going home to her other two children. But her newborn had to remain in our Nursery for seven days of I.V. antibiotic therapy. She will come to visit and

Beyond Nurses Notes

feed her infant every day and remember to take her own "Time Outs" for herself at home.

Mary M. Hale

Do You Want the Book Back?

I went in to check my patient and perform her assessment. I introduced myself and from under the covers comes a little voice, "Do you want the book back?"

Immediately, I remembered this patient from when she had been admitted to our floor as an ante-natal patient at 33 weeks gestation.

Joshua had been born naturally and was breast feeding and supplementing with Isomil. He weighed in at 5 pounds, 15 ounces and was very active and awake for feedings.

Mom was preparing for E.M.T. training and needed a book to help her. I gave her my Pediatric Advanced Life Support Review Book and told her she could keep it.

During the night her baby was in the Nursery and his body temperature dropped. We placed him under the radiant warmer.

In a few hours, his temperature was normal and he was feeding well.

When I told his Mother she said "Hypothermia, right?" She had studied the chapter in the PALS book.

Brian's Song

Jill was a 22-year-old first time Mom who delivered by Cesarean Section, after years of infertility treatment. Her joy was boundless. Brian's picture was on her wall.

Jill was an exceptional person herself. I got to know her as she came into our hospital as an outpatient for her ante-natal checkups. I would see her in the hallway almost three times a week and we got to know each other. When we finally met on our Post-Partum floor, she pointed to me and I pointed to her, and we both said, "What are you doing here?"

For the next four days we found out what we were doing here.

In 1998, as part of her past medical history, I found out she presented with headache, nausea, memory loss and fainting. At age 15 years, she had brain surgery for Arnold-Chairi malformation, which was caused by a disturbance during the period of her neural tube closure as an infant.

One of the major features of this malformation is displacement of part of the brain and fourth ventricle into the cervical canal.

At 36 weeks of gestation of the baby boy, Jill had a cesarean section to prevent any increased intercranial pressure to the brain.

At four feet, seven inches tall (170 pounds) Jill also had gestational diabetes. During her time with us, she continued to pump and take her breast milk to the Neonatal Intensive Care Unit to feed her infant. She was always faithful.

On the day of her discharge, I had promised her I

would stop in at 6:30am and say "Good bye and God bless," after I had worked all night in the Nursery.

When I opened her door after a soft knock, she was sitting her chair with her back to me, humming a lullaby to her son Brian's picture.

I didn't have the heart to disturb her. I called her later when I got home to wish her a safe trip and good luck!

Brian would remain in our NICU for another three weeks and then head home to Mom and Dad for Labor Day!

Beyond Nurses Notes

The Saga of the Boarder Babies

Who are you? You are babies of Mothers who have gone home and left you under our care for phototherapy which treats increasing bilirubin levels, or perhaps you are on a seven day course of I.V. antibiotic therapy.

But your "surrogate mother" is here doing your assessments, baths, and feeding you every three to four hours. Staff Nurses answer the phone when your Mom calls to inquire how you are doing.

Of course, she tells her how very special you are, the weight you have gained, and approximately how long you will stay with us.

Once one of you cries, it triggers your pals in the next crib to start, so we rotate your feeding schedule accordingly. We get into your rhythm.

I remember your Dad looking through the Nursery window at you under the warmer. His eyes wandered and saw me giving another baby his first immunization.

He called me over and asked what I was doing. I told him I was giving the baby's first immunization. He stated proudly that not one person in his family had ever been vaccinated. I explained to him how necessary it was and showed him a picture of my daughter, Maria, who was eight years old when she died of measles encephalopathy.

At the time of her death, the measles vaccine had not yet progressed from the lab.

He asked the Mother of his child and she agreed to the immunizations.

A lesson learned from the past.

Mary M. Hale

This Time Is All You Have

For those of us who have "seen the light," this world is never the same.

Most of you will not know what I am talking about. For the small number of you who have "coded," "crashed" in the Operating Room, or "thrown a clot" and became unconscious, your life is entirely different.

You are much more aware of the goings on around you. Small things that used to bother you don't bother you anymore. Family seems to mean a lot more to you. A fear that you will eventually lose your life does not bring any fear; in fact, deeply religious people welcome death in the future.

Sadness about leaving behind family, but, the joy of coming together with those family members who have gone before us, leaves us breathless.

The new life a baby brings to our family brings us HOPE.

The recognition of "This time is all you have" is wrapped around our brain, so say those patients interviewed post-resuscitation.

Our care in childbirth recovery is truly acute.

Thank you, Staff Nurses, for our lives.

Life Interrupted

Just as my book goes to the publisher, my physician gave me the diagnosis of uterine cancer (low grade, early stage). I thought about this for a few days and my blood pressure rose dramatically. For the first time in my life I had no control over something that I thought I could reduce with reason and relaxation breathing.

My pre-admission testing experience was filled with EKG, blood draws, x-rays and CAT scans. There was one bright light that stood out above the others – a physician's assistant anesthesiologist. She said I looked familiar as she took my history. I recognized her as a mother of an infant I had nursed in pediatrics with hyperbilirubinemia long ago. Her infant had very bad jaundice and was minutes away from an exchange blood transfusion. Due to her concern about her infant's condition, she could not go out for a bite to eat. She remembered that I brought her my peanut butter and jelly sandwich on whole wheat bread. She said that she often reminded her mother about the story. Then she said that my care for her did not stop there. She said that after the hospital phased out the pediatric floor, I transferred down to the maternity floor, where I nursed her with her second child on the postpartum floor.

Now I was the patient, imagine that! I often think of the article "Lessons I'm Leaving Behind" by Randy Pausch from the Philadelphia Inquirer Parade Magazine (Sunday, April 6, 2008). The themes that Randy presents are themes that I have tried to live my life by – "Always have fun," "Dream big," "Ask for what you want," "Dare to take a risk," "Look for the best in everybody,"

"Make time for what matters," and "Let kids be themselves." Remember, life can be interrupted for yourself.

When it comes to the finish line of life, most people accept that there may be failure, there may be disappointments, but the struggle is always gritty and measurable. Occasionally, if you are really lucky, something magical will happen.

Beyond Nurses Notes

References

1. Morse, RN, PhD, Janice M., "The Science of Comforting", <u>Reflections</u> – Sigma Theta Tau International Nursing Honor Society, 1996.

2. Pausch, Randy, "The Lessons I'm Leaving Behind", <u>Philadelphia Inquirer Parade Magazine</u>, 4/6/08 p. 6-7.

Other Publications by this Author

2009 **On Uganda's Terms** – 2nd edition, Hale, Mary M., RNC, MSN, CCB Publishing.

2005 **Maternity Matters – Vol. 1-2**
Stories by AEMC Maternity Nurses in process of publication.
To be incorporated into Dr. Sharon Hudacek's, Ph.D. book "Making a Difference: Stories from the Point of Care."

1998-2000 **Selected Tales from "The Comfort Basket" Published as Pediatric Chapter 5**
"Making a Difference: Stories from the Point of Care", Hudacek, Sharon PH.D, Center Nursing Press, A Division of Sigma Theta Tau International; Indianapolis, Indiana. pp. 60-69.

1997 **Dollops '97**, Vol. 4, No. 1, A Newsletter for Nurses, Provided by Astra USA,Inc., "Comfort Basket and EMLA Cream Help Take Away Pediatric Pain". Authors: Mary M. Hale, RN,C., MSN and June Lowe, RN,C.

1996 **Albert Einstein Healthcare Network, "A Nurse is a Rare Combination"** –
"Einstein Nurses…In Their Own Words" – "Tales from the Comfort Basket – The World of the Five Year Old" Author: Mary M. Hale, RN,C., MSN.

1995 **Nursing Times '95**, Albert Einstein Medical Center, "Crosstraining – A Journey of Rediscovery" Author: Mary M. Hale, RN,C., MSN.

1994 **Nursing Spectrum**, Vol. 3, No. 8, February 21, 1994: Nurse Entrepreneurs: "Clowning With a Difference" Authors: Tom Starner and Mary M. Hale, RN,C., MSN. An article about the beginnings of "Dear Lovely," the Delaware Valley's first Public Health – Teaching Clown for children and adolescents.

www.ingramcontent.com/pod-product-compliance
Lightning Source LLC
Chambersburg PA
CBHW022108160426

43198CB00008B/393